Everyday Clarity
with 52-Week Mental Health Guided Journal

Everyday Clarity
with 52-Week Mental Health Guided Journal

A Daily Wellness Companion to Reduce Stress, Boost Clarity, and Build Emotional Resilience All Year Long

Aria Capri Publishing
Devon Abbruzzese
Mauricio Vasquez

Authors:
Aria Capri Publishing
Devon Abbruzzese
Mauricio Vasquez

First Printing: July 2025

IISBN - 978-1-998729-59-3 (Hardcover Book)
ISBN - 978-1-998729-58-6 (Paperback)

FREE BONUS

Enjoy a Free Digital Copy of This Transformational Journal—My Gift to You

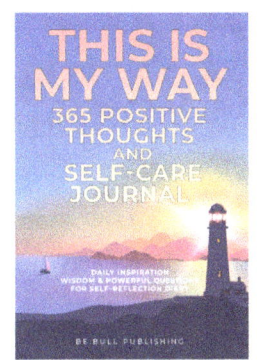

Thank you for showing up for yourself and taking this powerful step toward daily self-care, reflection, and personal growth.

As a heartfelt gift, I'm offering you a FREE digital copy of THIS IS MY WAY: 365 Positive Thoughts and Self-Care Journal.

It's packed with inspiring messages and thought-provoking questions to help you build confidence, reduce anxiety, and reconnect with what matters most —all year long.

Claim your free e-copy by scanning this QR code:

Prefer a Physical Copy?

Many readers love having a physical copy to hold, highlight, or gift to someone special. If that sounds like you, you can grab your printed copy here:

Buy the hardcover version on Amazon by scanning this QR code:

Thank you for allowing me to be a small part of your self-care journey.

Here's to a year of reflection, growth, and positive change.

A Small Favor That Makes a Big Impact

If this journal has helped you pause, reflect, reconnect, or grow in even the smallest way—I'd be deeply grateful if you'd consider leaving a review.

As an independent author, I rely on the honest words of readers like you to help others discover this book. Your feedback not only supports the continued life of this work—it also reminds me why these quiet moments of reflection matter, one person and one page at a time.

You can share your thoughts by scanning the QR code. It only takes a minute, but your words have the power to help someone else begin their own journaling journey.

Thank you, truly, for being part of this. Your time, voice, and support mean more than you know.

Devon

Want More Journals and Resources?

Whether you're enjoying this journal and want to explore more titles, or you're looking for a digital version you can use on your device, you've got options!

📚 Print On Demand Store – Physical Copies

Use this QR code to visit our Amazon store and order printed editions of our books.

📥 Gumroad Store – PDF Versions at a Lower Price

Scan this QR code to access our Gumroad store, where you can purchase downloadable PDF versions of our books at a lower price—perfect for printing at home or using digitally.

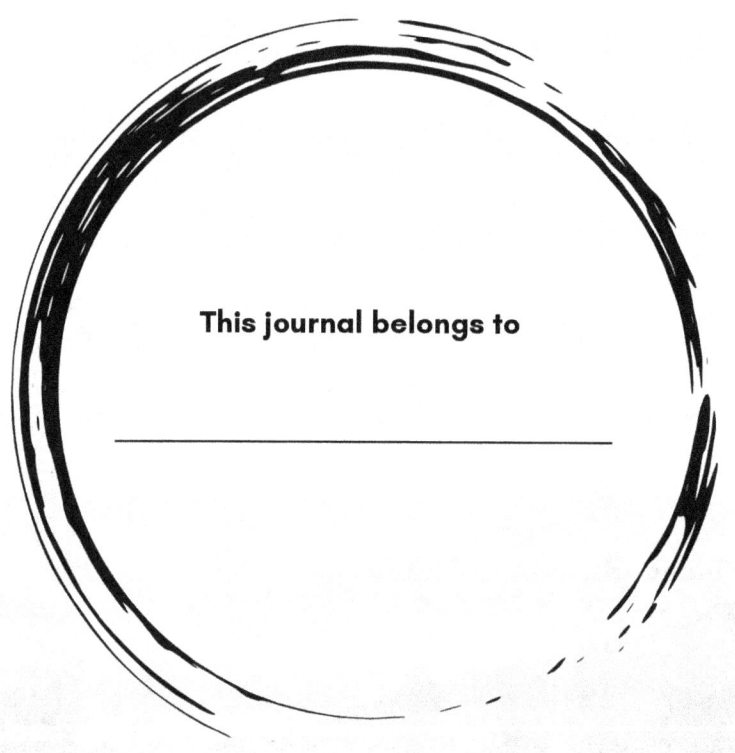

This journal belongs to

_____

Disclaimer

This journal is intended for personal reflection and general mental wellness support. It is not a substitute for professional advice, diagnosis, or treatment.

If you are experiencing emotional distress, a mental health crisis, or any situation that feels overwhelming, please seek guidance from a licensed physician, counselor, psychologist, or qualified mental health professional.

The author and publisher do not assume responsibility for any actions taken or not taken based on the content of this book. Use of this journal is entirely at the reader's discretion.

Your well-being matters—please reach out for professional help when needed.

Introduction

Welcome. You've just opened the door to something meaningful: a space designed for self-reflection, self-care, and steady emotional clarity. No matter where you're starting from—whether you're thriving, struggling, or somewhere in between—this journal meets you with care and without judgment.

Over the next 52 weeks, you'll be guided through daily prompts that explore the foundations of mental well-being. Each week follows a theme grounded in the four pillars of emotional and psychological resilience:

Calm and Resiliency, Connection and Engagement, Healthy Living, and Goals and Purpose.

These aren't abstract ideas. They're lived experiences—how you feel, relate, care, and grow. Journaling about them helps bring your attention back to what matters most: your inner life.

You don't have to write perfectly. You don't have to write a lot. Just write with honesty. Think of this as a small ritual—5 to 10 minutes of uninterrupted time each day to tune in, release what you're holding, and strengthen the connection to yourself. Whether you journal first thing in the morning, during your lunch break, or right before bed, consistency matters more than perfection.

Journaling isn't about fixing yourself. It's about staying curious. It's about becoming more aware of your thoughts, noticing your patterns, and creating a deeper sense of calm and clarity over time.

🌿 Calm and Resiliency

Stress is part of life—but how we respond to it can change everything.

This section focuses on building inner calm and bounce-back strength. Resilience doesn't mean never struggling; it means recovering thoughtfully.

Journaling here will help you notice the things that steady you, manage emotional turbulence, and foster self-trust even on difficult days. You'll explore simple practices for staying grounded—so you can face life's challenges with more steadiness and care.

🌷 Connection and Engagement

We all need meaningful relationships. But in a busy, digital world, connection can sometimes feel distant.

This section supports your emotional bonds with others and with yourself. These prompts are about recognizing the people who support you, reconnecting when you feel isolated, and exploring how relationships shape your sense of belonging.

They'll also guide you in building habits of engagement—like listening, sharing, and showing up with authenticity.

🌼 Healthy Living

How you care for your body shapes how you feel in your mind.

This section blends physical and emotional well-being—without perfectionism. You'll reflect on small daily choices that nurture you: sleep routines, nutrition, movement, digital boundaries, and self-kindness.

There's no one-size-fits-all path here. Instead, these prompts help you pay attention to what makes you feel more energized, present, and whole.

🌸 Goals and Purpose

You don't need a 5-year plan. You just need clarity about what matters today.

This section focuses on intention. You'll explore your values, your motivations, and the goals that energize you.

Whether you're rebuilding after burnout or reaching for something new, these prompts are designed to help you get unstuck, take ownership, and move toward purpose—even if it's one step at a time.

How to Use This Journal

Start any day you like. Keep this journal somewhere that feels inviting—your nightstand, your kitchen corner, your favorite chair.

There's no wrong way to journal. Write when you can. Skip a day if you need. Come back when you're ready. Your presence —not perfection—is what matters here.

Each daily prompt is short, supportive, and rooted in therapeutic insight. You'll find an easeful rhythm with time. And you may be surprised at how quickly you begin to feel clearer, steadier, and more emotionally connected.

This is your space to be honest, gentle, messy, quiet, bold— whatever you need today. There are no rules here, only invitations.

WEEK 1

Calm and Resiliency

1. If everything you deeply wanted came true by tomorrow, what would that feel like emotionally and physically?

....

....

....

....

....

2. Which of your heartfelt wishes feel possible with small steps or support?

....

....

....

....

....

3. What lights you up inside? How often do you give yourself permission to enjoy those moments?

....

....

....

....

....

4. Which inner strengths feel like gifts? How can you use them to nurture your well-being and purpose?

....

....

....

....

....

5. What calming words can remind you of your strength when life feels overwhelming?

....

....

....

....

....

6. What forms of care—emotional or practical—might make it easier to rise again after hardships?

....

....

....

....

....

7. What rituals help you feel held and rested as the week comes to a close?

....

....

....

....

....

Connection and Engagement

1. How do you nurture your relationships day to day, even during a busy week?

....

....

....

....

....

2. If someone who truly loves you could speak to you right now, what would they say? Write a few kind words to yourself.

....

....

....

....

....

3. Who do you turn to for support or laughter? What do those moments give you emotionally?

....

....

....

....

....

4. Who's been on your mind lately? What gentle step could you take to bridge the distance between you and them?

....

....

....

....

....

5. Recall a recent joyful moment with someone close. What filled you up about that experience?

....

....

....

....

....

6. If you wrote a heartfelt note to two close friends, what would you thank them for? How might it feel to send it?

....

....

....

....

....

7. What small, joyful or restful moment could you share with someone each day this week?

....

....

....

....

....

Healthy Living

1. What lifestyle changes would help you feel more whole, nurtured, or grounded?

....

....

....

....

....

2. What gentle step forward feels doable as you move toward those lifestyle changes?

....

....

....

....

....

3. What does physical care look like when it feels kind and intentional? How are you making space for that?

....
....
....
....
....

4. What's felt heavy or draining lately? What supportive actions or boundaries have you tried?

....
....
....
....
....

5. Think of a time when stress felt overwhelming. What do you remember feeling—both in your body and in your mind?

....
....
....
....
....

6. What helps you feel calmer when you're stressed? How does it change the way you feel?

....

....

....

....

....

7. As you slowly noticed your body from your feet to your head, what did you feel? How do you feel now?

....

....

....

....

....

Goals and Purpose

1. What hopes or intentions are you gently holding as you move through this journal?

....

....

....

....

....

2. What's a supportive action you could take to honor one of your hopes or intentions this week?

....

....

....

....

....

3. What did you imagine your future self becoming? What parts of that dream still live in you?

....

....

....

....

....

4. What gets in your way—and what beliefs or support systems keep you going?

....

....

....

....

....

5. In a role that aligned with your purpose, what would you be creating, leading, or nurturing?

....

....

....

....

....

6. If you could visit the past or future to grow, where would you go—and what would you hope to discover?

....

....

....

....

....

7. What gentle structure or ritual could support you in staying grounded and clear for the week ahead?

....

....

....

....

....

WEEK 5

Calm and Resiliency

1. What worry would feel lighter if you gave it a place to rest for now? Write it here, and come back when you're ready.

....

....

....

....

....

2. Pick a word that brings warmth or clarity. How does holding that word shift your attention and energy?

....

....

....

....

....

3. With each breath, what tension releases or emotion surfaces? What do you feel now?

....

....

....

....

....

4. What about your body and spirit feels beautiful or strong to you right now?

....

....

....

....

....

5. Think of a time when you rose after a fall. What did that moment teach you about your strength?

....

....

....

....

....

6. What connection would feel nourishing today—even if it's just a simple message or shared moment?

....

....

....

....

....

7. What small touches could turn your space into a sanctuary—one that supports your calm and healing?

....

....

....

....

....

Connection and Engagement

1. What kind of connection brings you joy and presence? What does that experience feel like?

....

....

....

....

....

2. Recall a connection that felt deep and real. What specific emotions did that connection bring to you?

....

....

....

....

....

3. Whose absence do you feel in your heart? What sweet, simple way could you reach out to them?

_____

_____

_____

_____

_____

4. Share a story of how one unexpected encounter became something meaningful in your life.

_____

_____

_____

_____

_____

5. What words of praise still warm your heart? What truth did they help you believe about yourself?

_____

_____

_____

_____

_____

6. What beautiful memories rise when you think of love, friendship, or laughter? What makes them so vivid?

....

....

....

....

....

7. Whose heart would light up from hearing from you? What honest and loving words would you share?

....

....

....

....

....

Healthy Living

1. Which self-care routines feel nourishing right now? How regularly do you lean on them?

....

....

....

....

....

2. What cozy or creative touches would turn part of your home into your own feel-good zone?

....

....

....

....

....

3. What five gentle habits would nurture both your body and spirit? What support might help you begin?

....

....

....

....

....

4. What gentle ritual or mindset shift could you begin today to invite more joy into your life?

....

....

....

....

....

5. Recall a moment of deep worry that ended up okay. What calming lesson would you carry into the future?

....

....

....

....

....

6. What changes—big or small—would make your space feel like a sanctuary for your well-being?

....

....

....

....

....

7. What small action could you take today to bring more harmony to your space—and what inspires you to do it?

....

....

....

....

....

Goals and Purpose

1. What dream still calls to you? What barriers—internal or external—have slowed your path?

....

....

....

....

....

2. What gentle weekly steps could bring your goal closer without overwhelm?

....

....

....

....

....

3. Is there a career or passion that still excites you? What's one small step you could take toward it today?

_____

_____

_____

_____

_____

4. If you could slip away for rest or inspiration, where would you go and how would it nourish you?

_____

_____

_____

_____

_____

5. If you wrote a love letter to your future self, what would you celebrate and affirm in her?

_____

_____

_____

_____

_____

6. What joyful, soul-nourishing experiences have you put off? How might you reclaim them gently?

....

....

....

....

....

7. What gentle structure or boundary could help you stay present and purposeful this coming week?

....

....

....

....

....

Calm and Resiliency

1. What kind of morning helps you feel your best? What's one small way you could bring more of that into your routine?

....

....

....

....

....

2. Which songs speak to your soul or body? What feelings do they help release or revive?

....

....

....

....

....

3. When anxiety or sadness passed, what wisdom did it leave behind for you to carry forward?

....

....

....

....

....

4. What activity brings calm to your heart or body? What sensations or feelings come with it?

....

....

....

....

....

5. Picture your favorite color surrounding you. What feeling or energy does it bring?

....

....

....

....

....

6. Imagine a sacred sunrise scene. What does your body feel, and what emotions come alive in you?

....

....

....

....

....

7. What helps you stay upright when life feels heavy? What rituals, thoughts, or support systems uplift you?

....

....

....

....

....

WEEK 10

Connection and Engagement

1. Picture a heartfelt gathering with loved ones. Who's there, and what makes the time together feel nourishing?

....

....

....

....

....

2. Who feels like a safe haven to you? What about their presence makes you feel seen and supported?

....

....

....

....

....

3. Who helped shape your confidence, growth, or sense of purpose? What do you carry from their influence?

....

....

....

....

....

4. What gentle kindness could you share this week, and how might that nurture your own spirit too?

....

....

....

....

....

5. What's one dream or experience you'd love to share with someone? Who would make it unforgettable?

....

....

....

....

....

6. If generosity had no limit, who would you pour it into—and what healing or hope would you offer?

....

....

....

....

....

7. What small act of service could you offer someone next week—and how might it soften or uplift you too?

....

....

....

....

....

Healthy Living

1. What nourishing foods feel both comforting and energizing? How can you savor them more often?

_____

_____

_____

_____

_____

2. How do your daily habits support your wellness? What gentle shifts would feel most loving to your body?

_____

_____

_____

_____

_____

3. What's your evening ritual or reward? Does it restore you—or is something else calling your body or heart?

....

....

....

....

....

4. Let your favorite place fill your senses. What comfort, clarity, or calm do you feel there?

....

....

....

....

....

5. When do you feel most at ease, radiant, or inspired during the day—and what are you usually doing then?

....

....

....

....

....

6. What drinks feel nurturing to your body or spirit? How might you make them part of a daily ritual?

....

....

....

....

....

7. What three calming actions feel most restorative when stress shows up in your body or mood?

....

....

....

....

....

Goals and Purpose

1. What do you need to feel balanced this week, and how can those needs align with your goals?

_____

_____

_____

_____

_____

2. What energy or vision has been quietly carrying you toward your goals recently?

_____

_____

_____

_____

_____

3. When you don't meet a goal, how do you speak to yourself?
What support do you wish you had in that moment?

....

....

....

....

....

4. What self-talk or thought habits make your path feel heavier
than it needs to?

....

....

....

....

....

5. What affirmations or practices help you break the cycle of
self-doubt or fear?

....

....

....

....

....

6. What are the soul-deep motivators that keep you walking forward, even on hard days?

....

....

....

....

....

7. What does success look like when it feels true to who you are? How would you describe it?

....

....

....

....

....

Calm and Resiliency

1. What calming song feels like a balm to your spirit? What message does it carry for you?

....

....

....

....

....

2. What helps you rise again after a hard moment—emotionally, physically, or spiritually?

....

....

....

....

....

3. What words of kindness do you need right now? Speak them to yourself with the care of someone who loves you.

....

....

....

....

....

4. What moment reminded you that you are stronger than you realized? What did you learn about yourself?

....

....

....

....

....

5. What kind of weather refreshes or soothes you? What outdoor activity brings you joy in that moment?

....

....

....

....

....

6. What's a sweet memory from childhood that still lights something inside you?

....

....

....

....

....

7. What item around you makes your heart smile? Describe the memory it's tied to.

....

....

....

....

....

Connection and Engagement

1. What kind of moments with friends feel the most nourishing or fun for you?

....

....

....

....

....

2. What heartfelt memory with a loved one still lingers in your mind and why?

....

....

....

....

....

3. What beautiful qualities in someone close feel empowering or touching to you?

....

....

....

....

....

4. Who offers you the kind of support your heart and mind need most? How have they shown up for you?

....

....

....

....

....

5. What wise or tender advice changed your path or perspective—and what came of it?

....

....

....

....

....

6. How might a dear friend describe your strength, presence, and spirit?

....

....

....

....

....

7. Who touched you with kindness this week? What small act of love or gratitude could you offer in return?

....

....

....

....

....

Healthy Living

1. What gentle body-based practices can you return to throughout the day to feel awake and balanced?

....

....

....

....

....

2. How did that breath and posture reset make your body or emotions feel different, even briefly?

....

....

....

....

....

3. How might drinking more water be a kind way to care for your body each day?

....

....

....

....

....

4. What's been affecting your sleep this week—and how might you gently support a better night's rest?

....

....

....

....

....

5. What calming habits could become your nighttime ritual— offering rest, softness, and renewal?

....

....

....

....

....

6. What dream made you feel bright or uplifted when you woke? What did it reveal or remind you of?

....

....

....

....

....

7. When your body or mood needs comfort, what drink do you reach for? What does it give you in that moment?

....

....

....

....

....

Goals and Purpose

1. What gentle, realistic goal could you set for yourself this week? How would it nourish or support you?

....

....

....

....

....

2. What brings you a deep sense of meaning or joy today? How does that connect to your evolving purpose?

....

....

....

....

....

3. If you had a space to help you stay organized and calm, what would it look like? How would it support you?

....

....

....

....

....

4. If resources were unlimited, how would you deepen your purpose—or protect what matters most?

....

....

....

....

....

5. If your heart could whisper one wish for more joy or peace, what would it ask for—and why?

....

....

....

....

....

6. What three goals feel important to your week—and what gentle actions will support their progress?

....

....

....

....

....

7. What aspects of your job or passion projects light you up? What makes them feel meaningful or fun?

....

....

....

....

....

Calm and Resiliency

1. Close your eyes and let a memory rise from a specific age. What does that memory reveal or stir in you?

....

....

....

....

....

2. Right now, do you feel more drawn to the ocean or the mountains? What do you think your heart is reaching for?

....

....

....

....

....

3. If you could gently change one past choice or moment, what would you hope to feel or understand differently now?

....

....

....

....

....

4. What kind of weather soothes your system—and how does it change your emotional state?

....

....

....

....

....

5. What songs help you feel powerful, alive, or radiant? Which ones do you return to when you need a lift?

....

....

....

....

....

6. What's flowing or stable in your life right now? What feelings does it bring to name that goodness?

....

....

....

....

....

7. What five things would feel joyful or kind to do next week? How can you make time for each one with care?

....

....

....

....

....

Connection and Engagement

1. Who surrounds you with joy, safety, or laughter? How do they awaken that feeling in you?

....

....

....

....

....

2. What would a beautiful, meaningful celebration for your dearest friend look like—and why that theme?

....

....

....

....

....

3. Who would you love to travel with on a meaningful getaway—and what shared joy would it bring?

....

....

....

....

....

4. What kinds of heartfelt or honest conversations make you feel deeply understood?

....

....

....

....

....

5. Are there any places nearby—like parks, cafés, or familiar spots —that feel joyful or meaningful when shared with others?

....

....

....

....

....

6. What live concert would fill you with excitement or healing—
and why that artist or group?

....

....

....

....

....

7. What five empowering or tender words describe someone you
love—and how do those qualities touch you?

....

....

....

....

....

Healthy Living

1. When you looked up at the sky, what feelings or thoughts came to you?

....

....

....

....

....

2. How do you see yourself—inside and out—and how gently can you move toward your ideal self-view?

....

....

....

....

....

3. If you were an athlete caring deeply for your body and mind, what would your routine include?

....

....

....

....

....

4. How did you feel—emotionally or physically—after your last walk, hike, or run?

....

....

....

....

....

5. How do eating and movement support or challenge your emotional and physical wellness?

....

....

....

....

....

6. What emotions rise when you think about food? What changes might bring more peace or joy to eating?

_____

_____

_____

_____

_____

7. What would a whole-hearted, healthy day look like—nourishing mind, body, and spirit?

_____

_____

_____

_____

_____

Goals and Purpose

1. When was the last time you lifted someone's spirit? How did that act of care feel to you?

....

....

....

....

....

2. What 10 loving or encouraging things could you do to uplift someone's heart or path?

....

....

....

....

....

3. What values, gifts, or moments do you want to live on in others after you're gone?

....

....

....

....

....

4. If you could only have health or wealth, which would you choose—and what emotion drives that choice?

....

....

....

....

....

5. What three small achievements would help you feel purposeful or proud this week?

....

....

....

....

....

6. What accomplishment still fills you with pride or gratitude—
and why?

....

....

....

....

....

7. What kind of museum visit would spark your curiosity or joy—
and who would you love to share it with?

....

....

....

....

....

Calm and Resiliency

1. What soothes your system when emotions run high—and how can you gently lean on those tools more often?

....

....

....

....

....

2. Without your phone for a day, how would you fill your time with connection, rest, or creativity?

....

....

....

....

....

3. What thoughts visited you during a quiet pause? What insight or emotions did they bring?

....

....

....

....

....

4. What helps shift your emotional energy when you're down—and what's the afterglow like?

....

....

....

....

....

5. Imagine a peaceful moment near water. What sounds, scents, and feelings wash over you?

....

....

....

....

....

6. Today I feel proud or peaceful within myself because... (What comes next?)

....

....

....

....

....

7. Recall a moment when you were scared but kept going. How did that shape your self-trust or strength?

....

....

....

....

....

Connection and Engagement

1. What fun or purposeful moments do you enjoy sharing with acquaintances or colleagues?

....

....

....

....

....

2. How would you like to show up or offer care in your local community in a way that feels authentic?

....

....

....

....

....

3. Walking the shore with someone dear—what would your heart or mind want to talk about?

_____

_____

_____

_____

_____

4. Who was the first person you called your best friend—and what did your time together feel like?

_____

_____

_____

_____

_____

5. What sensory or emotional experience did your last theater visit offer you? What made it special?

_____

_____

_____

_____

_____

6. What sweet or silly school memory sticks with you from childhood?

....

....

....

....

....

7. In your dream world of wonder, who travels with you—and how does the experience feel or unfold?

....

....

....

....

....

Healthy Living

1. Which language feels exciting to learn—and what dream or connection draws you to it?

....

....

....

....

....

2. What comforting or joyful show do you enjoy—and how does it help you reset or laugh?

....

....

....

....

....

3. If you sailed to a dream destination, what would bring you energy and delight on the journey?

....

....

....

....

....

4. Recall a time you felt grounded and vibrant. What were you doing to care for your whole self?

....

....

....

....

....

5. What do your favorite outfits make you feel—strong, free, good-looking? What do they say about you?

....

....

....

....

....

6. What do you often find yourself photographing—and how does it make you feel when you do?

....

....

....

....

....

7. What care rituals help you restore your energy after a demanding week?

....

....

....

....

....

Goals and Purpose

1. Picture your future five years ahead—what meaningful goals have you gently accomplished?

....

....

....

....

....

2. What emotions rise as you revisit one of your greatest accomplishments? What does it say about your growth?

....

....

....

....

....

3. What simple or deep gratitude is in your heart today? How does it soften or uplift you?

....

....

....

....

....

4. What kind of beauty, healing, or adventure would you seek on a planet where anything is possible?

....

....

....

....

....

5. What soulful or bold path would you take if money weren't a barrier—and who would you serve or uplift?

....

....

....

....

....

6. What message of gratitude would you share with a teacher who helped you grow?

....

....

....

....

....

7. If you followed your purpose across the map, where would you land—and how would you live?

....

....

....

....

....

Calm and Resiliency

1. What self-supportive tools help you navigate stress or hardship?

....

....

....

....

....

2. What sensations and emotions arise when you move through fear?

....

....

....

....

....

3. When fear makes something feel too hard, what words or actions help calm your inner voice?

....

....

....

....

....

4. When frustration arises, what's usually happening—and how do your thoughts react or spiral?

....

....

....

....

....

5. Recall a difficult day. What feeling weighed on you, and what gently shifted you toward healing?

....

....

....

....

....

6. What calming actions feel like medicine for your nervous system—and how long do they carry you?

....

....

....

....

....

7. When things don't go the way you hoped, what thoughts or feelings show up first?

....

....

....

....

....

6. If you could reconnect with someone from your past, who would it be—and what would you talk about or remember together?

....

....

....

....

....

7. What kind of soulful, fun, or romantic date would fill your heart with joy and connection?

....

....

....

....

....

Healthy Living

1. How is your energy across your thoughts, feelings, and body today—and what gentle support could lift each one?

....

....

....

....

....

2. Is your soul drawn to sunshine or soft gray skies? What feelings do they evoke in you?

....

....

....

....

....

3. What foods make you feel good—light, satisfied, or comforted?

....

....

....

....

....

4. What textures, colors, and items would turn your room into a healing retreat?

....

....

....

....

....

5. Which wellness space would support your energy and joy—a pool, court, or gym—and why?

....

....

....

....

....

6. If fear weren't holding you back, what would you feel ready to try? What part of you is eager to begin?

....

....

....

....

....

7. When your week flows well, how do you feel—and what habits or routines help make that happen?

....

....

....

....

....

Goals and Purpose

1. What inner voice or vision helps you move toward a goal with heart and hope?

....

....

....

....

....

2. What soothing, empowering steps support you when something scary stirs within you?

....

....

....

....

....

3. What healing gift would you offer for emotional pain—and why does that matter to your heart?

....

....

....

....

....

4. What past milestones still make you proud—and what inspired your steps?

....

....

....

....

....

5. What soul-aligned goal would bring you deep peace and pride if you achieved it in your lifetime?

....

....

....

....

....

6. What fears or patterns hold you back—and what compassion or clarity could help you move forward?

....

....

....

....

....

7. What loving message would you share with a friend who's unsure about chasing something big?

....

....

....

....

....

Calm and Resiliency

1. What beloved show feels like comfort or connection—and what does it offer you emotionally?

....

....

....

....

....

2. When anxiety whispers in specific situations, what self-compassionate steps do you take to soften it?

....

....

....

....

....

3. What triggered stress for you this week—and how can you support yourself if it happens again?

....

....

....

....

....

4. Write to your inner stress: "I see you, I've learned from you, and I'm choosing calm now."

....

....

....

....

....

5. What recent hurt or upheaval took energy—and how did you gently begin to heal?

....

....

....

....

....

6. Imagine a workspace that supports your happiness and wellness. What elements would it include?

....

....

....

....

....

7. What songs stir your spirit or remind you of your strength? What emotions or memories do they evoke?

....

....

....

....

....

Connection and Engagement

1. What five joys or passions might your closest friend have—and how well do you know her heart?

....

....

....

....

....

2. What would you pick with a gift card meant to brighten someone's day—and who comes to mind first?

....

....

....

....

....

3. If you had an unexpected day with someone inspiring, who would it be—and what heart-centered conversations might unfold?

....

....

....

....

....

4. What kind or powerful things do the people who support you do or say that remind you you matter?

....

....

....

....

....

5. What would bring joy, ease, or connection to a shared weekend with someone you love?

....

....

....

....

....

6. What words of healing or remorse would you offer with grace to someone you may have hurt?

....

....

....

....

....

7. What warm, vibrant, or inspiring day would you co-create with people around you?

....

....

....

....

....

Healthy Living

1. When your emotions feel heavy, what small comforts or activities bring relief?

....

....

....

....

....

2. Describe a lunch that leaves you feeling nourished and peaceful—what makes it special?

....

....

....

....

....

3. What helps you prepare meals that support both your body and mood?

....

....

....

....

....

4. What calming routines might help you drift off to a more peaceful sleep?

....

....

....

....

....

5. What are some ways you can move your body that feel joyful or freeing?

....

....

....

....

....

6. Picture a powerful version of you—what would she do, and how would she care for others?

....

....

....

....

....

7. Think of your inner superhero—what qualities could you start showing up with today, gently and with kindness?

....

....

....

....

....

Goals and Purpose

1. What's one thing that feels aligned or hopeful in your life today?

....

....

....

....

....

2. What's been tough lately? How can you reword that struggle with self-kindness or hope?

....

....

....

....

....

3. Picture something that warms your heart—what do you feel when you see it?

....

....

....

....

....

4. What gentle, consistent habits could keep your goals feeling aligned and achievable?

....

....

....

....

....

5. What does your dream day feel like? How could you intentionally shape your next day toward that?

....

....

....

....

....

6. What areas of your life are asking for growth—and how might you tend to them lovingly?

....

....

....

....

....

7. What small rituals or reflections help you savor your daily life more deeply?

....

....

....

....

....

Calm and Resiliency

1. Is there a place nearby that helps you feel calm, comforted, or recharged?

....

....

....

....

....

2. What room or place feels like a sanctuary—and how might you soften or beautify it further?

....

....

....

....

....

3. What keepsake in your space holds emotional or sentimental weight for you?

....

....

....

....

....

4. When you take a calm breath, what helps your heart or mind feel still and at ease?

....

....

....

....

....

5. When you're feeling truly happy, what kind of energy do others seem to notice in you?

....

....

....

....

....

6. Are there colors that make you feel peaceful—or ones that help you feel strong and confident?

....

....

....

....

....

7. After your last cry, how did your body or heart feel differently— what softened or settled?

....

....

....

....

....

Connection and Engagement

1. Who are your heart-friends? What about their personality brings you comfort or joy?

....

....

....

....

....

2. When sadness hits, who helps hold space for you? What do they offer that soothes you?

....

....

....

....

....

3. What gentle or joyful connections with others help lighten your mood when you're struggling?

....

....

....

....

....

4. What nourishing or playful activities would you love to do with a friend soon?

....

....

....

....

....

5. What dream feels possible with a little help? Who could walk beside you as it unfolds?

....

....

....

....

....

6. Who fills your heartspace—and how might you express love or gratitude to each of them?

....

....

....

....

....

7. Who's a friend from your past you miss? What caring words could reopen the door gently?

....

....

....

....

....

Healthy Living

1. How restful are your nights? What small changes could bring you closer to deep rest?

....

....

....

....

....

2. What task feels too heavy today? What would change if you gave yourself space from it?

....

....

....

....

....

3. How does the weather influence your emotional world? What shifts with each season or sky?

....

....

....

....

....

4. What creative or calming activity would you love to explore? What draws you to it?

....

....

....

....

....

5. What's been weighing on your heart lately? How might you take a small, caring step toward easing it?

....

....

....

....

....

6. What day lifts your spirit most? What do you often do that makes it feel special or supportive?

....

....

....

....

....

7. On a day like this, what activity brings comfort, creativity, or calm—and why?

....

....

....

....

....

Goals and Purpose

1. What's one small goal that would nourish or support you this week?

....

....

....

....

....

2. What affirmation lifts your spirit? How can you gently weave it into your days?

....

....

....

....

....

3. Is there a part of your life you wish to hold with more care—or more strength? What might that feel like?

....

....

....

....

....

4. If you could sit at a table with someone influential, what topic or vision or change would you talk about?

....

....

....

....

....

5. What would help your community feel safer, kinder, or more connected—and how might you help?

....

....

....

....

....

6. What would help you deepen your emotional closeness with the people who matter most?

....

....

....

....

....

7. What's calling you forward with a sense of hope or purpose as you look toward tomorrow?

....

....

....

....

....

Healthy Living

1. What calming rituals or reminders help you stay present when future thoughts feel overwhelming?

....

....

....

....

....

2. What gentle supports or boundaries help you soften anxious thoughts or stressful moments?

....

....

....

....

....

3. In times of deep fear, what brought you back to calm—or helped you hold on?

....

....

....

....

....

4. What difficult season showed you your strength, even when you weren't sure you had it?

....

....

....

....

....

5. What item in your wardrobe feels like emotional safety or softness to you? Why?

....

....

....

....

....

6. What kindness or gesture might offer someone in your world a sense of peace or safety?

_____

_____

_____

_____

_____

7. What joyful or tender experience this week lingers in your heart? What would it feel like to revisit it?

_____

_____

_____

_____

_____

WEEK 38

Connection and Engagement

1. Is there someone you miss being close to? What might you say or do to reconnect with them?

....

....

....

....

....

2. Who's your emotional anchor? What is it about them that brings comfort or security?

....

....

....

....

....

3. What was your last heart-to-heart about—and how did that moment connect you more deeply?

....

....

....

....

....

4. Do you lean toward joyful noise or comforting quiet in friendships—and what makes that feel good?

....

....

....

....

....

5. What connection-based activity helps soothe or spark you when you're feeling off?

....

....

....

....

....

6. What was the most heartfelt gift you've been given—and the one you've felt proud to give?

....

....

....

....

....

7. What silly or joy-filled story do you still laugh about when you remember it with a friend?

....

....

....

....

....

WEEK 39

Healthy Living

1. What five practices nurture your emotional and mental wellness?

....

....

....

....

....

2. Reflect on a time you felt emotionally taxed. What factors played a role?

....

....

....

....

....

3. What recent choice made you feel both healthy and joyful?

....

....

....

....

....

4. Which self-care practices from before still serve you today?

....

....

....

....

....

5. Who uplifts and inspires you? Imagine spending a day with them—what would you do?

....

....

....

....

....

6. What gentle reminders guide you toward self-care in tough times?

....

....

....

....

....

7. Which inner narratives might be limiting your self-care journey?

....

....

....

....

....

Goals and Purpose

1. What small shift today might bring more flow to your week?

....

....

....

....

....

2. What kind words can you offer yourself when things don't go as planned?

....

....

....

....

....

3. Which aspiration feels most aligned with your heart today?

....

....

....

....

....

4. Imagine your future self in two years. What's unfolding?

....

....

....

....

....

5. What wisdom would you pass on to someone chasing their dreams?

....

....

....

....

....

6. What nurturing elements can you weave into your daily flow?

....

....

....

....

....

7. What intention can you set for next week to feel more aligned?

....

....

....

....

....

Calm and Resiliency

1. What soothing practices help you navigate intense moments?

....

....

....

....

....

2. What boundaries can you set this week to care for yourself?

....

....

....

....

....

3. What changes can bring more serenity to your living space?

....

....

....

....

....

4. What kinds of situations tend to make you feel anxious, and what helps you feel calmer in those moments?

....

....

....

....

....

5. What no-cost pastime would uplift you tomorrow?

....

....

....

....

....

6. Take a moment to honor how you've gotten through hard times. What strength carried you forward?

....

....

....

....

....

7. What moments this week affirmed your self-worth?

....

....

....

....

....

Connection and Engagement

1. What practices deepen your self-love and acceptance?

....

....

....

....

....

2. What relational skills can you nurture to feel more connected?

....

....

....

....

....

3. What thoughtful actions could show your loved ones how much they mean to you?

....

....

....

....

....

4. What help can you provide to uplift someone else?

....

....

....

....

....

5. What moments with friends fill your heart with happiness?

....

....

....

....

....

6. How can you show up more fully in your friendships?

....

....

....

....

....

7. How can you and your close ones engage in collective self-care?

....

....

....

....

....

Healthy Living

1. What loving boundaries help you protect your time and energy?

....

....

....

....

....

2. How do you shield your emotional space from others who deplete your energy?

....

....

....

....

....

3. When did you feel your most vibrant? What self-care habits supported you then?

....

....

....

....

....

4. Imagine meals that make you feel cared for—what would they include?

....

....

....

....

....

5. What activities help you feel balanced, strong, and emotionally centered?

....

....

....

....

....

6. What grounding tools help you filter out negativity and stay true to yourself?

....

....

....

....

....

7. When you're seeking comfort, what nurturing choices could support you instead of turning to unhealthy choices?

....

....

....

....

....

Goals and Purpose

1. What does purpose feel like in your daily experience?

....

....

....

....

....

2. What defining moments helped you connect with your personal "why"?

....

....

....

....

....

3. What joy-centered goal could you bring to life this weekend?

....

....

....

....

....

4. What recent accomplishment reminded you of your strength or worth?

....

....

....

....

....

5. What have you done this week that you want to pause and celebrate?

....

....

....

....

....

6. Which short-term goal feels most aligned with your needs right now?

....

....

....

....

....

7. What's one gentle and powerful step you can take to move forward?

....

....

....

....

....

Calm and Resiliency

1. Where have you felt most soothed, safe, or seen? What stayed with you?

....

....

....

....

....

2. What bedtime practices bring you comfort and better rest?

....

....

....

....

....

3. What's a dream that felt healing, beautiful, or empowering?

....

....

....

....

....

4. What memory from this week brought you ease, joy, or lightness?

....

....

....

....

....

5. What inner strength helped you stay centered when things got hard?

....

....

....

....

....

6. Are there songs or lyrics that feel healing or comforting when you hear them?

....

....

....

....

....

7. What experience showed you that you're more resilient than you realized?

....

....

....

....

....

Connection and Engagement

1. What gentle gesture might bring more warmth or closeness to a relationship you value?

....

....

....

....

....

2. Is your heart carrying a hurt that's ready to heal? What would forgiveness look like for you?

....

....

....

....

....

3. What emotional space would forgiveness or boundary-setting create for you right now?

....

....

....

....

....

4. Who embodies the values you admire? How do those qualities speak to your growth?

....

....

....

....

....

5. Who are the loved ones you feel most thankful for right now? What have they brought into your life?

....

....

....

....

....

6. What small but thoughtful act could honor the people you're grateful for?

....

....

....

....

....

7. What community or cause speaks to your soul? What kind of support feels authentic to offer?

....

....

....

....

....

Healthy Living

1. What's making your to-do list feel heavy? How could you soften the load for your mind and body?

....

....

....

....

....

2. How do you nurture your emotional wellness alongside your physical care?

....

....

....

....

....

3. How are you really feeling right now—mentally, emotionally, spiritually? What would feel supportive?

....

....

....

....

....

4. What would it feel like to share your truth with someone who listens with care?

....

....

....

....

....

5. How would you talk to a friend about the value of seeking support when life feels heavy?

....

....

....

....

....

6. What feelings are sitting with you today? Which ones are speaking loudest?

....

....

....

....

....

7. Write a gentle note to your heart about why you deserve tenderness and care, every single day.

....

....

....

....

....

Goals and Purpose

1. What's different about your life now compared to a few years ago? What changes did you shape or survive?

....

....

....

....

....

2. What words do you return to when you need clarity, courage, or calm?

....

....

....

....

....

3. What's your emotional response when you face roadblocks on your path? How do you care for yourself then?

....

....

....

....

....

4. What insight about yourself has shaped your priorities or purpose this past year?

....

....

....

....

....

5. What story do you feel drawn to read or watch—and why might your heart need it right now?

....

....

....

....

....

6. What's one meaningful thing you'd love to do this weekend—and what could help you make it happen?

....

....

....

....

....

7. What form of giving back would light you up—and how might you start, even in a small way?

....

....

....

....

....

WEEK 49

Calm and Resiliency

1. What self-doubt are you ready to soften? What gentle step could help you let it go?

....

....

....

....

....

2. Describe a past experience of anxiety. What helped or would help you feel safer in that moment now?

....

....

....

....

....

3. If a close friend could respond to your worries, what comfort or insight might they give you?

....

....

....

....

....

4. How does your body respond to a few deep breaths? What sensations or emotions do you notice before and after?

....

....

....

....

....

5. What are you learning from your fears? What steps help you feel more secure or brave?

....

....

....

....

....

6. When fear speaks, how much of it reflects reality? What truths help soften the edges?

....

....

....

....

....

7. What calming rituals or practices have supported you through anxious moments? What else would you like to explore?

....

....

....

....

....

Connection and Engagement

1. What heart-centered actions can help deepen your connections with loved ones?

....

....

....

....

....

2. What gentle but firm boundaries could you set to care for yourself around others?

....

....

....

....

....

3. How does guilt affect your ability to say "no"? What helps you reclaim your voice with compassion?

....

....

....

....

....

4. What makes your presence nurturing or joyful for others—and how can you share more of that?

....

....

....

....

....

5. If you're facing a tough conversation, what can you do to feel calm and grounded beforehand? What might help you feel more prepared?

....

....

....

....

....

6. What heroine or story figure lights a spark in you? How could their traits show up in your real life?

....
....
....
....
....

7. What joy-filled or cozy activities would you love to plan with your loved ones soon?

....
....
....
....
....

WEEK 51

Healthy Living

1. What barriers stood in the way of your self-care or health goals this year?

....

....

....

....

....

2. How did you adapt or grow in the face of those health or emotional challenges? What worked?

....

....

....

....

....

3. How are you really feeling emotionally and mentally today? What's rising to the surface?

....
....
....
....
....

4. What self-nurturing routines do you want to carry into next year for body and mind?

....
....
....
....
....

5. How has journaling been a source of comfort, clarity, or empowerment for you?

....
....
....
....
....

6. What types of movement feel energizing or healing to you—and why?

....

....

....

....

....

7. What self-soothing strategies or boundaries can help protect your peace in the future?

....

....

....

....

....

WEEK 52

Goals and Purpose

1. Write a love note to yourself for your recent achievements. What makes them meaningful to your heart?

....

....

....

....

....

2. If you could manifest one soul-aligned goal next year, what would it be?

....

....

....

....

....

3. What's a nurturing first move you can make toward a goal that lights you up?

....
....
....
....
....

4. What transformations have taken root in you since the beginning of this journal? What are you proudest of?

....
....
....
....
....

5. What gentle affirmations feel like warm companions to carry with you daily?

....
....
....
....
....

6. What five growth moments or heart-wins are you celebrating at this journey's end?

....

....

....

....

....

7. Celebrate your soul's resilience. Write a heartfelt note to yourself honoring this year-long journey.

....

....

....

....

....

Keep Growing, Keep Asking: Discover More Titles

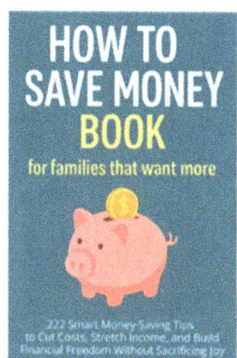

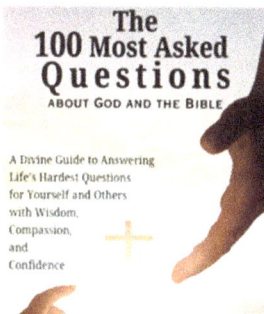

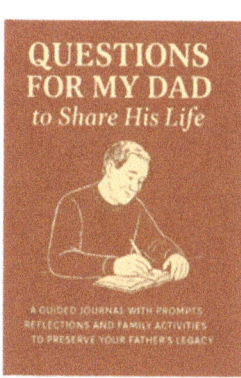

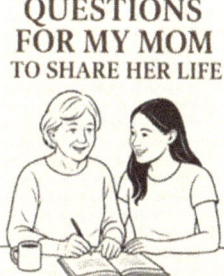

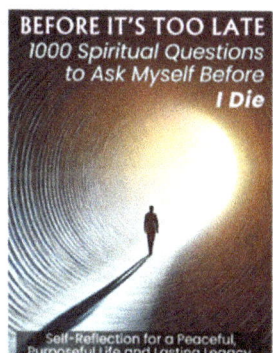

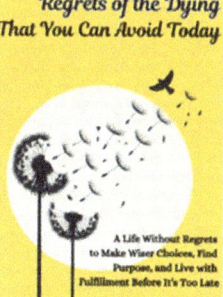